Published By Adam Gilbin

@ Charles Hester

Low Fodmap Diet: A Beginner's Step-by-step

Guide to Meal Plan for Better Health

All Right RESERVED

ISBN 978-1-990666-80-3

I0105874

TABLE OF CONTENTS

Low Fodmap Cup Of Noodles

Ingredients:

- 2 tablespoons freshly grated ginger

- 4 scallions, the green part chopped

- 1 jalapeno, thinly sliced

- 1 cup frozen carrots

- 1 cup tofu, drained and cubed

- 1/2 cup fresh basil, torn

- 3 cups cooked soba noodles (6 oz uncooked)

- ½ cup white miso paste (2 tablespoons is low fodmap)

- ¼ cup tamari

- 2 tablespoons sesame oil

- 1 tablespoon Texas Pete hot sauce

Directions:

1. Bring a large pot of water to boil and cook noodles according to package directions.
2. Drain and divide between the jars.
3. Combine the miso, tamari, sesame oil, hot sauce, and ginger in a medium bowl.
4. Divide this flavor mixture between the jars.
5. Divide the scallions, jalapeno, carrots, tofu and basil between the jars.
6. To serve, fill jar with hot water and allow to steep for about 2 minutes.
7. To store, cover with lids and chill for up to a week to eat at a later time.
8. When ready to serve, fill with hot water and allow to steep for about 2 minutes.

Gluten Free, Vegan And Fodmap Friendly 'Mince'

Lasagne

Ingredients:

For the 'mince':

- 2 tablespoons miso paste check that it's gluten free

- 3 tablespoons tomato paste

- 1 cup red wine or 1/2 water and 1/2 wine, although it won't be as flavourful

- 2-3 x 400g tins of plain tomatoes no added flavours (see notes)

- 2-3 medium carrots finely chopped

- 500 g tofu frozen the night before

- 2-3 tablespoons Tamari

- 2 tablespoons light brown sugar

- 2 tablespoons balsamic vinegar

For the 'cheese' sauce

- 5 cups plant based milk

- 2-3 tablespoons nutritional yeast

- 1 tablespoon light miso (i used shiro) optional, but adds cheesy umami

- 5 tablespoons vegan butter or olive oil

- 4 tablespoons gluten free cornflour (the starchy stuff, it might be called cornstarch where you live)

- Fine salt to taste

Optional:

- 1 teaspoon allspice

- 2 teaspoons dried sage

- 1-2 teaspoons dried rosemary

- 1 teaspoon oregano

- 1 teaspoon cinnamon

To finish:

- 2 packets gluten free lasagne sheets she's a big one

- Basil and spinach optional

- Vegan cheese, freshly grated

Directions:

To make the 'mince'

1. Add the olive oil to a large heavy bottomed saucepan over a medium heat. Once warmed, add the chopped carrot, and cook for about 15 minutes, or until it begins to shrivel and is starting to brown. While you're waiting, drain the tofu and tear it into small-ish mince like pieces.

2. Add the Tamari, light brown sugar and balsamic vinegar and stir really well to combine. Once the liquid volume has decreased, add the tomato paste and miso paste, and stir to combine.

3. Add the red wine to the pan, and stir well, collecting all the little browned bits at the bottom.

4. Next, add the tinned tomatoes, and stir thoroughly. Season with generous freshly cracked pepper, and follow with the tofu and herbs/spices, if you're using them.

5. Adjust the seasonings if necessary, and continue cooking for 10-15 minutes, until the tofu takes on some of the redness of the sauce, and looks like mince. You can add a bit of water to thin the sauce out, if necessary. If you're using the spinach and basil, you can mix it in here, or you can add it in the layering stage.

To make the white sauce:

6. While the mince is cooking, melt the vegan butter in a large saucepan. Once melted, add the cornflour, and whisk to combine until a paste forms.
7. Add the soy milk or plant based milk of choice. Once the mixture is smooth, add the nutritional yeast, miso and salt, adjusting for taste as you go.
8. Cook the white sauce for 10-15 minutes, until it is thick and spoonable.

To assemble:

9. Preheat the oven to 180 degrees Celsius or 356 Fahrenheit. Layer sheets of lasagne on the bottom of the baking dish. I used six and they fit perfectly, but this will depend on your dish size.

10. Follow this with half the 'mince' mixture, before adding another layer of pasta. Quickly follow this up with the white sauce (gluten free lasagne is quite dry and tends to curl up if you don't put something wet on top quickly.)

11. Lay more pasta on top of the white sauce, and quickly follow with the remaining mince. You can add another layer of pasta if you like, but because of the curling thing I like to spoon the white sauce right on top of the second layer of mince, and omit the last layer of pasta entirely.

12. Place the lasagne on a tray (to catch any overflow) and place in the oven for 30

minutes. You can serve warm, serve the next

day, or freeze for meals during the week

Warm Millet Porridge With Turmeric In Almond Milk

Ingredients:

- 1 cup of water or plant based milk

- 1/8 tsp ground vanilla

- rice malt syrup to taste

- 1/2 cup almond milk

- 1/2 cup millet

- 1 tsp coconut oil

- 1/2 tsp dried turmeric

- Toppings: Blueberries, cocoa nibs, bee pollen, pumpkin seeds, rice malt syrup

Directions:

1. Rinse 1/2 millet under warm water. In a small saucepan melt 1 tsp of coconut oil, add 1/2 tsp dried turmeric and roast for 10 seconds. Add millet.
2. For a nutty flavor, toast millet on medium heat for 2-3 minutes.
3. Add 1 cup of water or plant milk of your choice, 1/8 tsp of ground vanilla and sweeten to taste with rice malt syrup. Cook for 4-5 minutes.
4. Turn off heat, close with a lid and let sit for 10 minutes.
5. Warm and froth 1/2 cup of almond milk the help of a milk frother (like the one attached to espresso machines).
6. Scoop cooked turmeric millet into a bowl, pour over the frothed almond milk. Top with blueberries.

7. Sprinkle with crushed cocoa nibs, bee pollen, pumpkin seeds. Sweeten with more rice malt syrup if you like. Enjoy!

Low Fodmap Granola

Ingredients:

- 1 tsp cinnamon

- 1/2 tsp salt

- 1/4 cup | 2,37oz | 70ml maple syrup

- 1/4 cup | 2oz | 60ml melted coconut oil if solid, put in the microwave for 30 seconds

- 2 tbsp | 30g brown sugar

- 2 cups | 7oz | 200g rolled oats gluten free if intolerant

- 1/2 cup | 1,75 oz | 50g walnuts

- 2 tbsp | 20g flax seeds

- 2 tbsp | 20g pumpkin seeds

Directions:

1. Preheat oven to 300ºF/ 150ºC.

2. Measure oats, walnuts and seeds into a big bowl.

3. Add the maple syrup, sugar and oil and stir until well blended.

4. Spread out the mix on a large baking sheet lined with parchment paper.

5. Bake for 40 minutes or until the oats are golden brown and fragrant, and gently stir with a spatula every 10 minutes.

6. Let the granola cool completely in the baking tray and store it in an airtight container for up to 2 weeks.

Chicken Enchiladas

Ingredients:

From-scratch enchilada sauce

- 2 tsp of red chili powder

- 2 cups of low-FODMAP chicken stock

- ½ tsp of salt

- ½ tsp of cumin

- ½ tsp of oregano

- 1 medium-sized saucepan

- ¼ cup garlic-infused oil (OR ¼ cup of onion infused oil)

- 415 g of diced tomatoes - canned

- ¼ cup of all-purpose flour (gluten-free)

Actual enchiladas

- ¼ tsp of red chili powder

- 10 corn tortillas

- 115 g of fresh green chilies

- 1 cup of sharp cheddar cheese (can use extra sharp cheddar cheese)

- 200 g of feta cheese

- ½ tsp of salt

- ½ tsp of cumin (can use more to taste)

- 1 large mixing bowl

- 1 large nonstick skillet

- 1 small plate

- ½ tsp of oregano (can use more to taste)

- 1 small mixing bowl

- 1 oven-safe glass dish (13 x 19 inches, or something equivalent)

- Freshly ground black pepper

- 680 g of boneless, skinless chicken breast

- 1 cup of Havarti cheese

- 2 tsp of garlic-infused oil (OR 2 tsp of onion infused oil)

- ¼ cup of cilantro

- ½ cup of green onions/scallions (only use green part)

Directions:

1. First, we will begin by preparing the red enchilada sauce from scratch.
2. Take your saucepan, and set it over a medium flame.
3. Add in your oil and let it heat quite a bit in the pot.
4. At this point, add in your flour a little at a time and whisk while it mixes in and cooks with the oil for about a minute or two. This will help cook out the raw flour taste from the finished sauce.
5. Once that is lightly cooked, whisk in your chili powder and stir for about 30 seconds. Then, slowly begin to add the rest of the INGREDIENTS: in the following order: chicken stock, canned diced tomatoes, cumin, salt, and oregano.

6. Stir these INGREDIENTS: together to mix well, and then let the mixture sit in the pot and come to a light boil.

7. Let the sauce simmer and heat thoroughly for about 10 minutes and then remove from heat and set aside. This Directions: will make about 3 cups of sauce. You are free to use this entire quantity for the enchiladas, but if you don't need it all, you can store it in the fridge in a covered container for up to 2 weeks.

8. As the sauce is simmering for those 10 minutes, you can begin preparing the enchiladas. Start by dicing the chicken into smaller pieces and place them into your large mixing bowl. Add the cumin, salt, oregano, chili powder, and black pepper to taste into the mixing bowl with the chicken. Toss the chicken chunks to coat them completely with all these spices.

9. Put your large non-stick skillet over a medium flame, and add the oil you have chosen for the enchiladas.

10. Heat the oil and then add the coated chicken pieces into the pan. Let the chicken cook for about 3–5 minutes until it is just beginning to lose its natural pink color or when it is halfway cooked.

11. At this point, the from-scratch red sauce should be ready to take off the heat.

12. Add in a splash of this into the pan with the chicken, along with your minced green chilies, and fully coat the chicken in this.

13. Continue cooking the chicken in the pan for another 3–5 minutes until it is completely cooked and heated all the way through.

14. Now, you can prepare the oven that has been preheated to 350 degrees Fahrenheit. Use a rack when cooking this dish in the oven, and place it in the middle of your oven. Coat the

bottom of your baking dish with a little bit of your enchilada red sauce.

15. Now, place your shredded cheddar and Havarti cheeses into a small mixing bowl, and mix them evenly. On a small plate, set one corn tortilla down and coat its entire surface with the red sauce.

16. Place a small amount of cooked chicken down the middle of the tortilla and lightly sprinkle some cheese from the small mixing bowl on top.

17. Roll up the tortilla and place it, face down, into your oven dish.

18. Repeat this process until you have used up all the corn tortillas, all the chicken, and about 1/3 of the shredded cheese mix.

19. Again, you can choose how much red sauce to use for each step in this recipe. Place all the tortilla rolls close together in the oven dish.

20. Pour a good amount of the remaining enchilada sauce over the rolled tortillas in the oven dish and distribute the remaining cheese (about 2/3 of the starting amount) over the rolled tortillas. Evenly crumble the feta cheese over the top and bake for about 20–30 minutes. Remove the dish from the oven once the enchiladas have cooked and the cheese is golden brown and bubbly.

21. Finally, top the baked dish with your finely chopped scallions and cilantro, and divide the dish into 6 even servings.

22. Eat one and share or save the rest. Enjoy!

Pumpkin Carrot Risotto

Ingredients:

- 1 and ½ of cup uncooked risotto rice

- ½ cup of leeks (only use the green tips)

- 1 tbsp of garlic-infused oil

- 4 cups of a low-FODMAP vegetable stock

- 4 cups of spinach leaves

- 1 roasting tray or pan

- 1 large saucepan

- 240 g of Japanese pumpkin (OR sweet potato or buttercup squash)

- 2 and ½ of tbsp lemon juice

- 2 large carrots

- Salt and pepper

- 2 tsp of lemon zest

- 3 tbsp of fresh cilantro

- 1 tbsp of olive oil spread OR dairy-free butter

- 1 tbsp of olive oil

- 50 g of parmesan cheese (OR vegan soy-based cheese)

Directions:

1. Begin by preheating your oven to 390º F.
2. Peel the skin off the carrots and pumpkin.
3. Chop them into small, even-sized pieces and distribute them evenly on a roasting tray, coating with olive oil.

4. Dust some pepper and salt, according to your preference.
5. Bake the veggies for 25 minutes at most or until they begin to look soft and the color is golden brown.
6. Make sure to toss the veggies a couple of times as they cook.
7. Add your dairy-free spread and garlic-infused oil into a large saucepan and cook roughly chopped leeks in the pan for 2 minutes over medium heat.
8. Add your uncooked risotto rice to the pot and stir for a minute.
9. Pour the vegetable stock, gradually (a half cup at each time) until the rice cooks and absorbs all the liquid. Lower the heat as the rice cooks more and more to avoid any of it sticking to the bottom of the pot.

10. As the rice finishes cooking, add in your shredded spinach, salt, pepper, lemon juice, and lemon zest.
11. Finally, stir in the baked pumpkin and carrot pieces and top with chopped fresh cilantro and the cheese of your choice.

12. Serve in a bowl while hot and enjoy!

Salad Niçoise

Ingredients:

- 1 teaspoon Dijon mustard

- Pinch of sugar

- 3 (about 250g each) tuna steaks

- 12 cherry tomatoes, halved

- 100g (2/3 cup) kalamata olives

- 12 (about 650g) baby potatoes

- 320g green beans, topped

- 4 eggs

- 60ml (1/4 cup) extra virgin olive oil

- 1 tablespoon red wine vinegar

- 1 cup fresh parsley leaves

Directions:

1. Cook the baby potatoes in a saucepan of boiling water for 10 minutes or until tender.
2. Transfer the potatoes to a chopping board and chop them coarsely.
3. Add the beans to the pan and cook until bright green. Run under cold running water to stop the cooking process.
4. Dip into ice water to crisp the beans so they will be crunchy. Drain well.
5. Hard boil the eggs, peel and slice.
6. Whisk together the mustard, oil, vinegar and sugar in a bowl or small blender.
7. Sprinkle liberally with salt and pepper.
8. Heat a grill to medium-high heat. Add the tuna and cook for 2-3 minutes each side for medium or longer if you prefer.
9. Place to the side and let it rest for at least 5 minutes.

10. Lightly slice the tuna vertically to place onto the salad for eye appeal.

11. Divide the potato, green beans, egg, tuna, tomato, olives and parsley among the serving bowls.

12. Drizzle the dressing over the tuna and salad. Season with salt and pepper to serve.

Savory Chicken And Rice Muffins

Ingredients:

- 1 1/3 cups grated fresh mozzarella cheese

- 3 green onions, thinly sliced, the green tops only

- 1/4 cup basil leaves, chopped finely

- 3 eggs, lightly beaten

- 2/3 cup Basmati Rice

- 250g skinless smoked chicken breast, chopped finely

- 2/3 cup dried tomatoes, coarsely chopped

Directions:

1. Preheat oven to 400F. Grease Texas sized muffin tin. Line the muffin tin with liners.
2. Cook the basmati rice as the package suggests. Rinse the rice and let cool.
3. Place all INGREDIENTS: into a bowl, with the exception of 1/3 cups of the mozzarella cheese.
4. Spoon the mixture of chicken and rice into the prepared muffin pan.
5. Sprinkle with remaining cheese. Bake for 15 to 20 minutes or until the muffins are firm and light golden in color.
6. Stand in pan for 5 minutes. Dump the muffins onto a plate and allow to cool. Store in an airtight container.
7. Refrigerate until ready to serve. Enjoy for breakfast or as a light tea snack.

Spiced Baked Potato

Ingredients:

- ¼ teaspoon sea salt

- ½ teaspoon paprika, smoked

- ¼ teaspoon black pepper

- ½ teaspoon garlic-infused oil

- 4 cups potatoes, sliced

- 4 eggs

- ¼ cup olive oil

- ½ teaspoon curry powder with turmeric

Directions:

1. Place potatoes in a bowl together with spices. Drizzle with olive oil and mix well.
2. Wrap 1 cup of potatoes with foil. Repeat step with remaining potatoes.
3. Put the foil packs in a tray and bake for 30 minutes in a preheated oven at 400 degrees Fahrenheit.
4. Remove tray from the oven. Open each foil pack slightly and crack an egg on top.
5. Cook in the oven for another 10 minutes.

Frozen Cranberry Smoothie

Ingredients:

- 1 cup cranberries, frozen

- 1 tablespoon lemon juice

- 4 oz. coconut milk

- 10 oz. orange juice

- 1 firm banana, sliced

- 1 teaspoon pure maple syrup

Directions:

1. Place all of the INGREDIENTS: in a food processor.
2. Blend until smooth.

Low Fodmap Hearty Kale Sausage Soup

Ingredients:

- 2tbs garlic injected olive oil

- 1-2 bundles kale, deveined and hacked

- 4 cups Low FODMAP broth

- Squeeze red pepper drops

- Squeeze fennel seeds

- Add Salt and Pepper to taste

- 1lb Low FODMAP wiener, any packaging removed

- 2 enormous carrots, destroyed

- 4 enormous yukon gold potatoes, skin on, diced

- 1/2c lactose free milk/cream

Directions:

1. Start by caramelizing the hotdog in a huge soup pot on medium-high warmth. Evacuate and deplete on paper towels.
2. Include the garlic imbued oil, destroyed carrots, the red pepper pieces, a shake of salt, and a couple of toils of dark pepper. Let those cook for around 10 minutes on medium-low warmth, blending as often as possible.
3. When the carrots get delicate and build up some shading, hurl the frankfurter back in, alongside the potatoes and the stock. Give it a decent mix and afterward let it cook on medium-low warmth for around 40 minutes, or until the potatoes are as delicate as you can imagine them.
4. Include the kale, and permit to cook for another 5-10 minutes with a cover on, so the kale gets pleasantly steamed. If you decide to

make it a more extravagant dish, presently would be an ideal opportunity to include the drain or cream, give it a decent mix and appreciate!

Low FODMAP Veggie Fritters With Lime Basil Sauce

Ingredients:

- 2 eggs

- 1 tsp sweet paprika

- 1 tsp genuine salt

- ½ tsp crisply ground dark pepper

- Vegetable oil for cooking

- 1 little zucchini/courgette, ground

- 2 little potatoes, ground

- ¼ cup green onion, green part just, hacked

- 2 cups breadcrumbs

Lime basil sauce

- ¼ cup Low FODMAP acrid cream

- 1 tbs Low FODMAP mayonnaise

- 1 tbs lime juice

- 1 tbs crisp basil, cleaved

- 1/2 tsp garlic imbued oil

- Salt and pepper to taste

- Side Salad

- 3 cups blended spring greens

- ¼ cup carrot, stripped and ground

- ¼ cup regular tomato, diced

- 2 tbs sunflower seeds

Serving of mixed greens dressing

- 1 tbs additional virgin olive oil

- Run of unadulterated maple syrup

- Salt and pepper to taste

- 1 tbs lime juice

- 1 tbs garlic implanted oil

Directions:

1. Start by grinding the potato and zucchini, flushing the shreds with cool water, and crushing out as a lot of fluid as you can. Lay the shreds on a buildup free kitchen towel.

2. Prep the remainder of the waste fixings and combine them in a huge blending bowl.

3. Coat the base of a griddle with vegetable oil and warmth on medium high. Structure the

waste blend into patties and sauté until
brilliant on each side.

4. While you're singing the wastes, combine the
    elements for the Lime-Basil Sauce in a little
    holder and put in a safe spot.

5. For the side serving of mixed greens, I simply
    toss the dressing fixings in a bricklayer
    container, seal the top firmly and shake it - at
    that point use tongs to disperse dressing
    equally over the greens. Top with carrot,
    tomato and sunflower seeds.

6. Serve and enjoy yourself!

Speedy Spaghetti Bolognese

Ingredients:

- 2 teaspoons garlic-infused olive oil

- 2 pounds (900 g) extra-lean ground beef

- 8 ounces (225 g) lean bacon slices, diced

- 2-⅔ cups (670 ml) tomato puree

- 2 teaspoons cayenne pepper

- ½ teaspoon chili powder (optional)

- Two 12-ounce (350 g) or three 8-ounce (225 g) packages gluten-free spaghetti

- 2 teaspoons olive oil

- Salt and freshly ground black pepper

- Grated Parmesan, for serving

Directions:

1. Bring a large pot of water to a boil.
2. Add the spaghetti and cook according to package directions, until just tender.
3. Drain, return to the pot, and cover to keep warm.
4. Meanwhile, heat the olive oil and garlic-infused oil in a large heavy- bottomed frying pan over medium heat.
5. Add the beef and bacon and cook until the beef is nicely browned, breaking up any lumps as you go.
6. Add the tomato puree, cayenne, and chili powder (if using) and simmer for 10 minutes, stirring occasionally.
7. Season to taste with salt and pepper.
8. Divide the spaghetti among four bowls and spoon the Bolognese sauce over each.

9. Garnish with Parmesan and serve immediately.

Penne With Meatballs

Ingredients:

- 1 large egg, beaten

- 2 teaspoons garlic-infused olive oil

- 2 teaspoons olive oil

- 3 to 4 heaping tablespoons finely chopped basil

- ¼ cup (15 g) finely chopped flat-leaf parsley

- ½ teaspoon cayenne pepper

- Salt and freshly ground black pepper Olive oil, for pan-frying

- 2 pounds (900 g) extra-lean ground beef

- 1 cup (220 g) cooked long-grain rice

- ¾ cup (60 g) grated Parmesan

- One and a half 12-ounce (340 g) packages gluten-free penne (18 ounces/510 g total)

- 2 cups (500 ml) tomato puree

- ¼ cup (5 g) roughly chopped basil

- Grated Parmesan, for serving

- Extra basil leaves, for serving (optional)

Directions:

1. Bring a large pot of water to a boil.
2. To make the meatballs, combine the beef, rice, Parmesan, egg, garlic- infused oil, olive oil, finely chopped basil and parsley, cayenne, and salt and pepper in a large bowl.

3. With wet hands, shape into golf ball–size balls.

4. Heat the olive oil in a large frying pan over medium heat, add the meatballs, and cook until nicely browned on all sides and cooked through.

5. Meanwhile, add the pasta to the boiling water and cook according to package directions until just tender. Drain, return to the pot, and cover to keep warm.

6. Pour the tomato puree over the meatballs and sprinkle on the roughly chopped basil. Bring to a boil, then reduce the heat and simmer for 2 to 3 minutes, until warmed through.

7. Divide the penne among four bowls and spoon the meatballs and sauce over the top. Garnish with a sprinkling of Parmesan and extra basil leaves, if desired, and serve immediately.

Chocolate Pavlova With Pomegranate, Raspberries & Kiwi

Ingredients:

Meringue:

- 4 - large egg whites & ¼ - teaspoon cream of tartar

- 1 - cup (198 g) sugar, preferably superfine

- 2 teaspoons cornstarch & ½- teaspoon apple cider vinegar

- ½ - teaspoon vanilla extract

- 4 - ounces (115 g) bittersweet chocolate, finely chopped, preferably at least 60 to 70% cacao

Topping:

- 12 - raspberries, very firm and fresh

- 2 - green kiwi, peeled and sliced crosswise into thin rounds

- 1 - cup (240 ml) heavy cream, chilled

- 2 - teaspoons confectioners' sugar & 3 - tablespoons pomegranate seeds

Directions:

1. For the Meringue: Preheat broiler to 250°F/121°C. Line a preparing sheet field with material paper and follow a 9-inch (23 cm) hover on the paper; turn paper over.

2. Dissolve the chocolate until easy and allow to chill to scarcely heat; installed a safe spot.

3. In a great, oil-free bowl whip egg whites with inflatable whip connection of stand blender or utilize an electric powered mixer on low speed till foamy.

4. Include cream of tartar and hold beating, going tempo to high, till delicate pinnacles shape. Include sugar slowly and beat till meringue is hardened and reflexive so that you can take a few minutes.

5. Beat in cornstarch, vinegar, and vanilla.

6. Sprinkle the chocolate over the meringue and in all respects tenderly make more than one folds to deliver chocolate streaks in the course of the meringue.

7. You can OVER blend in all respects effectively. Decide in want of much less.

8. Scoop the meringue onto fabric inside the circle and make use of the returned of a giant spoon to assist shape a spherical plate in the drawn circle, being aware so as not to exhaust the marbling.

9. Make a moderate sorrow inside the focal factor of the circle.

10. You will hear the whipped cream and natural product inside the middle and a downturn within the meringue will assist hold the fixings.

11. A spot in stove and heat for 1 hour 15 minutes, at that point, test the meringue circle.

12. It ought to be sparkling, dry and simply tinged with the faintest degree of shading.

13. Keep heating for 15 minutes more if essential. Mood killer stove and enable the plate to chill inside the broiler.

14. Once cooled, the plate is probably put away in a water/air evidence compartment at room temperature for as long as 3 days.

For the Toppings:

15. Whip the cream in a clean and calm bowl with the sugar until the shape of a touchy pinnacle. spot meringue circle on level presentation platter.

16. Heap the whipped cream inside the focal point of the meringue, permitting a fringe of meringue to stay. spot natural product over whipped cream, to a wonderful quantity, and serve in (chaotic) wedges with spoons to scoop the whole thing up.

Mediterranean Fish Stew With Garlic Toasts

Ingredients:

- 200ml white wine

- 350ml fish stock

- 3 strips orange zest

- 1kg skinless halibut fillets, cut into large
  chunks

- 500g clams

- 400g large raw prawns

- handful flat-leaf parsley , chopped

- For the garlic toasts

- 1 large ciabatta loaf, cut into 1cm slices

- 5 tbsp olive oil

- 3 tbsp olive oil

- 1 large onion , sliced

- 2 garlic cloves , sliced

- 1 red chilli , finely chopped

- 2 tbsp tomato purée

- 1kg tomatoes , roughly chopped

- 2 garlic cloves , halved

Directions:

1. To make the garlic toasts, drizzle the bread with oil, then griddle or grill until golden all over.

2. While the toasts are still hot, rub them with garlic and set aside.

3. Heat the oil in a wide, deep frying pan.

4. Add the onion and cook over a gentle heat for 5 mins until softened.

5. Stir through the garlic and chilli and cook a couple of mins more.

6. Add the tomato purée and tomatoes.

7. Turn up the heat and cook for 10-15 mins, stirring until the tomatoes are pulpy.

8. Pour over the wine and cook for 10 mins more until most of it has boiled away.

9. Add the fish stock and orange zest and heat until gently simmering.

10. Nestle the halibut chunks into the liquid and cook for 5 mins.

11. Add the clams and prawns and cook for 5 mins more until the fish is cooked through and the clams have opened (discard any that haven't).

12. Sprinkle the parsley over the stew and serve with the garlic toasts.

Easiest Ever Paella

Ingredients:

- 300g long grain rice

- 1l hot fish or chicken stock

- 200g frozen pea

- 400g frozen seafood mix, defrosted

- 1 tbsp olive oil

- 1 leek or onion, sliced

- 110g pack chorizo sausage, chopped

- 1 tsp turmeric

Directions:

1. Heat the oil in a deep frying pan, then soften the leek for 5 mins without browning.
2. Add the chorizo and fry until it releases its oils.
3. Stir in the turmeric and rice until coated by the oils, then pour in the stock.
4. Bring to the boil, then simmer for 15 mins, stirring occasionally.
5. Tip in the peas and cook for 5 mins, then stir in the seafood to heat through for a final 1-2 mins cooking or until rice is cooked.
6. Check for seasoning and serve immediately with lemon wedges.

Poached Eggs On Toast

Ingredients:

- A slice or two of gluten-free bread

- 1 tbsp butter (or non-dairy version)

- 2 fresh eggs

- 1 tbsp. of white wine vinegar

- Salt and pepper

Directions:

1. Add the vinegar to a pan of hot water and let it boil at a slow, gentle simmer.
2. Prepare your bread for toasting.
3. Stir the water with a spoon so that a whirlpool is created in the centre of the pan and gently slide your eggs one at a time into the whirlpool.

4. Poach for 3-4 mins, depending on how soft you like your eggs, toasting and buttering your bread in the meantime.

5. Remove the eggs from the water with a slotted spoon and drain on a piece of kitchen towel.

6. Place on top of your toast and season with salt and pepper.

Scrambled Eggs

Ingredients:

- Salt and pepper

- 2 slices of gluten-free bread

- 2 eggs

- 1 tbsp butter (and some for buttering your toast)

Directions:

1. Put your slices of bread in the toaster ready to go for when you're ready and have your butter at hand too.

2. Place the tablespoon of butter in a saucepan and add your eggs.

3. Put the saucepan over a low to medium heat and beat the eggs so they become liquid.
4. Slowly cook the eggs, stirring all the while, until they start to solidify.
5. Make your toast in the meantime and butter it when ready.
6. Once the eggs are cooked, but still slightly loose, pour them on top of your buttered toast, season with salt and pepper and eat.

Fodmap Friendly Pumpkin Soup

Ingredients:

- 1 teaspoon light brown sugar

- Pinch of salt

- Freshly cracked black pepper

- Pinch of cinnamon

- Pinch of chilli flakes I used Aleppo

- 3 cups stock

- 2 tablespoons peanut butter optional

- 1.5 kg piece of Kent or Japanese pumpkin it will be around 1.2kg after skin is removed

- 3 tablespoons olive oil

- 20 g+ peeled and chopped ginger

- 1/2 – 1 teaspoon asafoetida powder optional (mimics garlic and onion flavour)

Directions:

For a roasted pumpkin soup:

1. Preheat the oven to 200C or 400F and line a baking tray.
2. Cut the pumpkin into larger pieces, leaving the skin on. Rub the skin with 1 1/2 tablespoons of olive oil and place it on the baking tray, skin side up, and into the oven. Bake until cooked though (this will depend on how large the pieces are but budget for around an hour or more). Once cooked, remove the skin and proceed with the ginger cooking step.

For a regular pumpkin soup:

3. Cut the pumpkin into even cubes. I find slightly larger cubes easier to blend at the end if you're using a stick blender.

4. Preheat the oil in a large soup pot over a low-medium heat. Add the ginger and cook for a couple of minutes until fragrant. Add the sugar, asafoetida powder and cinnamon (or any spices/woody herbs you're using) and cook a minute more until they're fragrant, too.

5. Add the pumpkin pieces and stir to coat. Add the 3 cups of stock and stir again to pick up any caramelised bits from the bottom of the pot. I recommend leaving it at 3 cups of stock and adjusting at the end if you prefer a thinner soup – a thick soup can be corrected but a thin soup is a lot harder to fix. On that note, wait to salt the soup until the end when the flavours have melted and you can determine how salty it is already.

6. Cook for 10-15 minutes for the roasted pumpkin soup, and 20-30 for the regular. Keep in mind that the secret to a good soup is uniformly cooked vegetables that will blend smoothly (without leaving thin watery bits and chunky pumpkin bits) so don't rush the cooking process.

7. When the pumpkin is completely cooked, take it off the heat. Add the peanut butter, if you're using it. Using whatever blending tool you have on hand, blend the soup until smooth. Adjust for seasoning, and add a little extra liquid (plant milk, regular milk, cream or stock) if you want a thinner soup.

8. Keep in mind: a Nutribullet doesn't have a steam escape valve so you can't blend a hot soup in one. I recommend a stick (immersion) blender for soup, because you have a lot of control and can season it as you go. That said,

you could also use a Vitamix if you have one (I don't).

9. To finish, garnish with whatever you fancy (I used crème fraiche, Aleppo chilli oil, honey toasted pepitas and lemon zest because I'm a wanker) and serve.

10. Keeps well in the fridge for a few days and also freezes well.

Gluten-Free Dijon Baked Chicken Fingers

Ingredients:

- 1 tablespoon olive oil

- 1/4 cup Dijon mustard

- 2 garlic cloves minced

- 2 eggs

- 1 pound boneless skinless chicken breast cut into strips

- 3 cups gluten-free cornflakes preferably organic, non-GMO

- 1/2 teaspoon paprika

- 1/2 teaspoon sea salt

Directions:

1. Preheat the oven to 425 degrees F. Line a baking sheet with parchment paper.

2. In a small food processor, pulse the cornflakes with the salt and paprika until finely ground. Remove to a shallow bowl and drizzle in the olive oil. Whisk with a fork until the cornflake crumbs are coated and not clumping together.

3. In a second bowl, beat the eggs until smooth.

4. In a large mixing bowl, combine the Dijon and garlic. Add the chicken and toss until well coated.

5. Working one by one, dredge the chicken in the cornflake mixture, shaking off any excess. Dip the tenders in the egg and return them to the cornflakes, pressing down until fully coated. Arrange the tenders in an even layer on the baking sheet.

6. Bake in the oven until golden and crispy, 15 to 20 minutes. Allow to cool slightly on the tray, then serve alongside ketchup and mustard.

Paleo & Low Fodmap Sweet And Sour Chicken

Ingredients:

- 2 tablespoons coconut oil

- 1/2 cup (100 gram) coconut sugar or regular white sugar

- 1/4 cup (60ml) apple cider vinegar

- 2 tablespoons Coconut Aminos, or gluten free soy sauce/tamari

- 1/4 cup (60 g) ketchup or Low FODMAP Ketchup

- 1/4 cup (60 ml) chicken stock

- 1 red pepper cut into chunks

- 1 cup (65 g) pineapple chunks

- 1 pound boneless, skinless chicken breasts, cut into 1-inch chunks

- 1/2 cup (65 grams) arrowroot starch or cornstarch

- 1 large egg beaten

- 3 spring onions stalks, green part only for low fodmap

Directions:

1. First prepare the sauce by adding the coconut sugar, vinegar, coconut aminos, chicken stock and ketchup to a medium sauce pan. Stir and bring to a boil. Reduce to a low heat and leave until later.

2. Add chicken pieces and beaten egg to a large ziplock bag. Seal and shake to coat chicken. Then add the arrowroot starch to the bag,

shaking again to lightly coat all the chicken pieces.

3. Add coconut oil to a large non skillet. Add the coated chicken. Fry over medium heat, a couple of minutes on each side until the coating begins to crisp. Add pepper and pineapple chunks. Continue to saute over medium heat until chicken is browned and cooked through.

4. Add the sauce to chicken and peppers. Cover and reduce the heat down to a simmer and allow the juices to soak into the chicken for a few minutes. Top with sliced green onions. Serve over rice and enjoy!

Fennel Carrot Soup

Ingredients:

- 3 cups of a low-FODMAP vegetable stock

- 1 tbsp of garlic-infused oil

- 1 tbsp of olive oil spread OR dairy-free butter

- 1 and ½ tbsp of fresh cilantro

- ½ cup of a low-FODMAP milk

- 1 tbsp of olive oil

- 8 slices of a low-FODMAP bread

- 1 large saucepan

- 1 blender/food processor

- 2 large carrots

- 200 g of sweet potatoes

- 340 g of regular potatoes

- ½ cup of leeks (only use the green tips)

- Salt and pepper

Directions:

1. Begin by thinly slicing the green tips of the leeks. Peel the potatoes, carrots, and sweet potatoes and then chop them into small chunks.

2. Warm a large saucepan using a low flame, and pour both the olive oil and garlic-infused oil.

3. When it's warm enough, cook the sliced leeks, stirring occasionally. They cook fast—about a minute—so watch out.

4. After this, add the potatoes, sweet potatoes, and carrots into the saucepan and cook on low for about 5 minutes.

5. Continue stirring the contents of the saucepan.

6. Turn the flame under the saucepan to medium, and add the vegetable stock.

7. Allow the soup to boil and then cover the saucepan. Let it simmer for not more than 15 minutes or until the veggies are soft.

8. While the soup is simmering, melt the dairy-free spread in a frying pan, where you heat the fennel seeds for about a minute while stirring.

9. Add in freshly chopped cilantro and stir together for another minute.

10. Add this fennel and cilantro mixture to the soup.

11. Pour the soup out of the large saucepan, and allow it to cool for about 10 minutes once the vegetables are fully tender.

12. Then, pour the soup into a blender and process until the soup is smooth and looks more or less homogenous.

13. Pour the soup mixture back into a saucepan and begin reheating it over a low flame.

14. Mix in your low-FODMAP milk and make sure to season with salt and pepper.

15. Top the soup with fresh cilantro and a side of lightly toasted low-FODMAP bread. Enjoy!

Lentil And Rice Bowl

Ingredients:

- 400 g of canned lentils

- Salt and pepper

- 3 cups of low-FODMAP vegetable stock

- 240 g of Japanese pumpkin (OR sweet potato or buttercup squash)

- 1 tbsp of olive oil

- 1 and ½ cups of uncooked long-grain brown rice

- ½ tsp of smoked paprika

- ¼ cup of green onions/scallions (only use green part)

- 3 large carrots

- Juice of 0.5 large lime

- 1 and ½ cups of baby spinach leaves

- 1 red chili - mild

- 1 pinch of chili powder

- ½ cup + 3 tbsp of fresh cilantro

- 2 tsp of garlic-infused oil

- 1 large saucepan

- 1 roasting pan or tray

- 2 cups of frozen edamame beans

- 1 small saucepan

- 1 large frying pan

- 1 blender/food processor

- 1 tsp of ground cumin

- 3 tbsp of lightly toasted pumpkin seeds

Directions:

1. Begin by preheating your oven to 390º F.
2. Place the rice into a large saucepan over a medium flame, add in your vegetable stock, and bring the contents of the saucepan to a rolling boil.
3. When it has started to boil, cover the pot, and reduce the flame.
4. Allow the rice to simmer for 20 minutes.
5. Add another 10 minutes when the water has not fully evaporated.
6. Peel and cut the pumpkin and carrots to your desired size; ideally, they have to be small pieces.

7. Coat the pumpkin and carrot chunks in olive oil, salt, and smoked paprika, and place them in a roasting tray.

8. Bake them for up to 30 minutes until they appear golden brown, making sure to toss the veggies once as they cook.

9. Roughly chop the chilies, spinach, and green onions, making sure to deseed the chilies first.

10. Place them in the blender, along with garlic-infused oil, ½ cup cilantro, and 3 tbsp of water.

11. Blend the INGREDIENTS: into a chunky paste and then stir in with the brown rice while it cooks.

12. Once the rice is finished, let it stand for 10 minutes and then fluff the rice, adding some salt and pepper according to your preference.

13. Set a frying pan over medium flame on the stove.

14. Drain and rinse the canned lentils and add them to the pan.
15. Add the cumin and chili powder, as well as the quarter cup of water to the pan and simmer for a maximum of 5 minutes or until the water has been incorporated into the lentils.
16. Remove the lentils from the heat and place them on the side.
17. Add some lime juice and some more salt and pepper, if you wish
18. Boil the frozen edamame beans in a saucepan until they are tender.
19. In a serving bowl, plate the spiced rice and lentils, and top it with edamame, roasted veggies, pumpkin seeds, and the remaining cilantro. Enjoy!

Smoked Salmon Appetizers

Ingredients:

- 1 egg yolk

- 140g smoked salmon, plus extra for gnoshing

- 1 tbsp chopped parsley

- 2 tbsp gluten-free flour mixed with 1 tsp coarsely ground pepper

- Oil, for frying

- 2 large baking potatoes

- 2 tbsp olive oil

- Grated zest and juice ½ lemon

- Grape tomatoes, for garnish

Directions:

1. Microwave potatoes on high for 10-12 mins until fork tender. Let cool for 5 mins, scoop out the insides into a bowl, smash with a fork and flavor with olive oil, a sprinkle of lemon juice and the zest, and then add the egg, salmon and parsley.

2. Shape into small cakes with a large tablespoon and place in the fridge to chill.

3. Sprinkle each cake with the peppered flour, then fry over a low heat in a little oil for 2-3 mins on each side.

4. Drain on a paper towel. Serve warm with a halved grape tomato and parsley for color.

Spinach And Butternut Squash Salad

Ingredients:

- 1 tablespoon fresh lemon juice

- 4 tsp brown sugar

- 2 tablespoons extra virgin olive oil

- 2 teaspoons wholegrain mustard

- 1 x 150g pkt baby spinach leaves

- 600g butternut squash, peeled and sliced into bites

- 2 teaspoons olive oil

- 2 teaspoons honey

- 2 teaspoons sesame seeds

- 1 x 75g pkt toasted pine nuts

Directions:

1. Preheat oven to 425F. Line a baking tray with parchment paper.
2. Place the pieces of squash in a bowl, drizzle with the oil and 3 tsp of the brown sugar. Sprinkle with salt and pepper.
3. Place the squash onto the baking tray and into the oven.
4. Bake for 25 minutes or until golden brown, turning once during cooking. Remove from the oven and sprinkle evenly with the sesame seeds.
5. Return to the oven and bake for 5 minutes or until the seeds are lightly toasted. Remove from the oven and set aside for 30 minutes to cool.
6. Combine the lemon juice, olive oil, mustard and extra honey in a small blender and whir until well combined.

7. Season with salt and pepper.

8. Place all the INGREDIENTS: into a serving
    bowl.

9. Drizzle with the dressing and gently toss until
    just combined. Serve immediately.

Peanut Butter Baked Oatmeal

Ingredients:

- ½ firm banana, mashed

- 60 milliliters almond milk, unsweetened

- 15 grams peanut butter

- 40 grams oats

- Salt

Directions:

1. Place banana in a bowl together with milk and oats. Mix well and season with salt.
2. Transfer the mixture to an oven dish. Put peanut butter in the center and cover with mixture.
3. Cook for 15 minutes in a preheated oven at 180 degrees Celsius.

Cucumber Sesame Salad

Ingredients:

- 1 sweet pepper, chopped

- 1 tablespoon sesame seeds

- 1 teaspoon kosher salt

- 2 tablespoons rice vinegar

- 1 tablespoon sesame oil

- 1 tablespoon lime juice

- 2 seedless cucumbers, grated

- 2 tablespoons cilantro, chopped

- 2 carrots, grated

- 1 green onion leaves, sliced

- 1 tablespoon pure maple syrup

- 1 tablespoon soy sauce, gluten-free

- 1 teaspoon ginger, grated

Directions:

1. Sprinkle salt over cucumbers to remove excess liquid. Set aside for 15 minutes.

2. Place rice vinegar, sesame oil, lime juice, ginger, soy sauce, and maple syrup in a bowl. Mix well to create dressing.

3. Put cucumber together with sweet peppers and carrots in a separate bowl. Drizzle with prepared dressing and toss to coat.

Maple-Marinated Salmon With Sesame-Spinach Rice

Ingredients:

- (4-oz) salmon filets, skin evacuated

- Cooking shower

- 1 3/4 cups water

- 1/2 to 3/4 tsp genuine salt (to your taste)

- 2 cups moment dark colored rice

- 4 cups infant spinach leaves

- 1 tbsp toasted sesame seeds

- 1 tbsp dim/toasted sesame oil

- 1/4 cup garlic-imbued oil

- 1/4 cup unadulterated maple syrup

- 2 tbsp sans gluten soy sauce or tamari (I utilized low-sodium)

- 1/4 tsp crisply ground dark pepper

- 4 scallion tops, cut

Directions:

1. In a medium bowl, whisk together the garlic oil, maple syrup, soy sauce and dark pepper.
2. Spot salmon filets in an enormous compress top pack and include garlic-maple blend. Hurl to cover and refrigerate for 2 to 4 hours.
3. Preheat broiler to 400F. Line an enormous, rimmed preparing sheet with thwart and fog with cooking shower.
4. Spot salmon on a heating sheet and shower a touch of the marinade over the top.

5. Heat until salmon is hazy in the thickest part and arrives at 145F on a moment read thermometer, 12 to 18 minutes, contingent upon thickness.

6. In the meantime, heat the water and salt to the point of boiling in a huge pot.

7. Mix in rice and come back to bubbling.

8. Lessen warmth to low, spread, and stew for 5 minutes. Expel from warmth and rest, secured, 5 minutes more.

9. Fog an enormous nonstick skillet with cooking shower and warmth to medium-high.

10. Include spinach and cook until shriveled.

11. Lessen warmth to low and include rice, sesame seeds and sesame oil (If your skillet is too little to even think about fitting all the rice, add the spinach to the pot with the rice).

12. Hurl tenderly to cover, separation rice among 4 plates and top with salmon.

13. Enhancement with scallions and serve.

Pesto Pasta With Grilled Chicken And Roasted Tomatoes

Ingredients:

Broiled tomatoes

- 16 cherry tomatoes, split

- 1 Tbsp. garlic-mixed olive oil

- Flame broiled Chicken

- 4 little chicken bosoms

- 1 Tbsp. garlic-mixed olive oil

- 1 tsp. dried oregano

Pasta

- 8 oz. uncooked without gluten pasta (like rotini or penne)

Pesto

- 2 (0.75 oz.) bundles new basil

- ¼ cup chives

- ¼ cup pine nuts

- ½ lemon, juice of

- ¼ cup garlic-mixed olive oil

- Salt and pepper, to taste

Directions:

1. Preheat the stove to 350°F. Hurl cherry tomato parts with olive oil and spread equitably onto a shallow preparing container. Cook until skins are wrinkled and marginally caramelized; around 30 minutes. Put in a safe spot.

2. Preheat the tabletop flame broil. Spot chicken bosoms, olive oil, and oregano in a huge bowl and hurl to blend. Flame broils chicken until done. Permit to cool marginally before cutting. Put in a safe spot.

3. Prepare pasta as indicated by bundle guidelines.

4. Meanwhile, place basil, chives, pine nuts, lemon juice and olive oil in a blender. Mix until smooth.

5. Once pasta is cooked, deplete and flush before coming back to pot. Add pesto to pasta and mix until pasta is well-covered. Top with cooked tomatoes and cut barbecued chicken.

6. Season to taste with salt and pepper and serve warm.

Seafood Pasta With Salsa Verde

Ingredients:

- 2 small squid bodies, cleaned and sliced into rings

- 8 ounces (225 g) boneless, skinless firm white fish fillets, cut into cubes

- 1 pound (450 g) raw large shrimp, peeled and deveined, tails intact

- 1 pound (450 g) fresh shelled mussel meats

- ½ cup (125 ml) light cream

- 2 tablespoons plus 2 teaspoons dry white wine

- 1 pound (450 g) gluten-free pasta

- ½ cup (130 g) Salsa Verde

- 2 teaspoons olive oil

- 2 teaspoons garlic-infused olive oil

- Salt and freshly ground black pepper

Directions:

1. Bring a large pot of water to a boil. Add the pasta and cook according to package directions, until just tender. Drain and return to the pot. Stir in most of the Salsa Verde, cover, and keep warm.

2. Meanwhile, heat the olive oil and garlic-infused oil in a large nonstick frying pan over medium-high heat. Add the squid, fish, and shrimp and cook for 2 minutes, tossing gently. Stir in the mussel meat, cream, and wine, reduce the heat, and simmer for 3 to 4

minutes, until all the seafood is lightly cooked
through. Season to taste with salt and pepper.

3. Divide the pasta among four bowls and spoon
    the seafood sauce over each. Finish with small
    dollops of the remaining Salsa Verde and
    serve immediately.

Smoked Chicken Pasta

Ingredients:

- 10 ounces (285 g) boneless, skinless smoked chicken breast or plain roast chicken breast, sliced

- 2 large handfuls of baby spinach leaves, rinsed and dried

- ⅓ cup (50 g) pine nuts

- ½ cup (40 g) grated Parmesan

- 1 pound (450 g) gluten-free pasta

- ¼ cup (60 ml) extra virgin olive oil

- 2 teaspoons garlic-infused olive oil, plus more for serving (optional)

- Salt and freshly ground black pepper

Directions:

1. Bring a large pot of water to a boil.
2. Add the pasta and cook according to package directions, until just tender.
3. Drain and return to the pot. Stir in 2 tablespoons of the olive oil, cover, and keep warm.
4. Heat the garlic-infused oil and the remaining 2 tablespoons olive oil in a large frying pan.
5. Add the chicken, spinach, and pine nuts and cook, stirring, until the spinach has wilted and the chicken and pine nuts are golden brown.
6. Add the drained pasta and Parmesan and toss over medium heat until the cheese has melted.
7. Season to taste with salt and pepper and finish with an extra drizzle of garlic-infused oil, if desired.

Simple Low Fodmap Potato & Egg Salad

Ingredients:

- 1 - small cucumbers & 3 - tbsp fresh chives

- 3 - tbsp green onions/scallions & 85ml (1/3 cup) mayonnaise

- 1 - tbsp lemon juice & 1 - tbsp wholegrain mustard

- 800g – potato & 160g - green beans

- 4 - large egg & 1 - red bell peppers

- Season with black peppe

Directions:

1. Clean and cut the potatoes into reduced down pieces (strip if important). Set up the inexperienced beans with the aid of reducing

into little portions. Spot the potatoes in an great pot and spread with water. Spot the top of the pan and deliver the water to a moving bubble over medium-high warmness. At that point flip down the warmth to medium-low and permit to bubble for 15 to twenty minutes till the potatoes are delicate. Add the inexperienced beans to the pan, around 3 minutes earlier than you channel the potatoes.

2. Enable the inexperienced beans to cook dinner for two to three mins, until sensitive and splendidly shaded.

3. Channel and notice to the other side to cool.

4. While the potatoes cook dinner, hard-warmness up the eggs.

5. Spot the eggs in a bit pot of water and spread with virus water.

6. Spot the pot over medium-excessive warmth and bring the water to a transferring bubble.

7. Permit to bubble for 2 minutes earlier than turning the warmth all the way down to the maximum minimal warmth placing. Cook for 10 to twelve minutes.

8. Channel and run the eggs under virus water before stripping. Cut the eggs into quarters.

9. While the eggs cook dinner, installation the cucumber and pink chile peppers.

10. Strip the cucumber and cut into off sticks.

11. Deseed and bones the red chime peppers.

12. Finely scale back the inexperienced onions/scallions (inexperienced pointers just) and chives.

13. Make the serving of blended veggies dressing by means of combining the wholegrain mustard, mayonnaise, lemon juice and numerous drudgeries of darkish pepper.

14. In an enormous bowl tenderly integrate the potatoes, inexperienced beans, difficult-bubbled eggs, cucumber, crimson chime

peppers, green onions/scallions (fresh hints just), chives and plate of combined greens dressing.

15. Season with two or three drudgeries of dark pepper.

Maple And Sesame Chicken With Brown Rice

Ingredients:

- pinch salt & ½ - tsp vegetable oil

- 1 - tsp black sesame seeds & 1 - tsp sesame seeds

- a - handful of fresh coriander leaves

- 1 - tsp pumpkin seeds, chopped

- 4 - tsp maple syrup & 4 - tsp gluten-free soy sauce

- 450g/1lb - boneless, skinless chicken thighs & 150g/5oz - brown rice

To serve

- 1 - tbsp sesame oil & 1 - tbsp rapeseed oil

- 2 - heads of bok choi, halved

Directions:

1. In a bowl, combine the maple and without gluten soy sauce. Include the chicken thighs and blend until totally covered in the marinade.
2. Spot the blanketed chook thighs into a chilly, profound, overwhelming based pot.
3. Spot the dish onto a medium warmth and cook dinner until the hen is cooked via and the nectar and soy covering has thickened to a reflexive coating.
4. In the meantime, including rice, 300ml/10½fl oz. Water, and salt to a special container and produce to the bubble.
5. When the water is effervescent, decrease the warmth and stew the rice, secured, until delicate.

6. For the bok choi, warmness the sesame and rapeseed oil in an extensive griddle over medium warmth.

7. Include the bok choi and cook dinner for three-5 mins, or until the leaves have contracted.

8. At the point when the rice is cooked, cushion it with a fork, at that point blend through the oil, sesame seeds, and coriander. Sprinkle over the slashed pumpkin seeds.

9. Make use of spoon to serve the rice onto serving plates and pinnacle with the hen. Spot the bok choi close by.

Chicken And Mushrooms

Ingredients:

- 50g cubetti di pancetta

- 300g small button mushroom

- 2 large shallots, chopped

- 250ml chicken stock

- 1 tbsp white wine vinegar

- 50g frozen pea

- 2 tbsp olive oil

- 500g boneless, skinless chicken thigh

- Flour, for dusting

- Small handful parsley, finely chopped

Directions:

1. Heat 1 tbsp oil in a frying pan. Season and dust the chicken with flour, brown on all sides. Remove. Fry the pancetta and mushrooms until softened, then remove.
2. Add the final tbsp oil and cook shallots for 5 mins.
3. Add the stock and vinegar, bubble for 1-2 mins.
4. Return the chicken, pancetta and mushrooms and cook for 15 mins. Add the peas and parsley and cook for 2 mins more, then serve.

Zesty Haddock With Crushed Potatoes & Peas

Ingredients:

- 1 tbsp capers, roughly chopped

- 2 tbsp snipped chives

- 4 haddock or other chunky white fish fillets, about 120g each (or use 2 small per person)

- 2 tbsp plain flour

- 600g floury potato, unpeeled, cut into chunks

- 140g frozen peas

- 2 ½ tbsp extra-virgin olive oil

- Juice and zest ½ lemon

- Broccoli, to serve

Directions:

1. Cover the potatoes in cold water, bring to the boil, then turn to a simmer.
2. Cook for 10 mins until tender, adding peas for the final min of cooking.
3. Drain and roughly crush together, adding plenty of seasoning and 1 tbsp oil. Keep warm.
4. Meanwhile, for the dressing, mix 1 tbsp oil, the lemon juice and zest, capers and chives with some seasoning.
5. Dust the fish in the flour, tapping off any excess and season. Heat remaining oil in a non-stick frying pan.
6. Fry the fish for 2-3 mins on each side until cooked, then add the dressing and warm through.
7. Serve with the crush and broccoli.

Egg In A Cup With Buttered Toast

Ingredients:

- Salt and pepper to taste

- 2 slices of gluten-free bread

- 2 eggs

- 1 tbsp. of butter (or non-dairy version), but you can use more if tolerated.

Directions:

1. Put the eggs in a saucepan filled with cold water and bring it to the boil. (If you put the eggs straight into boiling water they'll probably crack.)
2. Put your toast in the toaster in readiness for when the time comes.

3. Boil the eggs for 7=8 mins and then drain them.

4. Taking care because the eggs will be hot, peel off the shells of the eggs and place the eggs in a bowl.

5. Make your toast.

6. Add the butter to the eggs and mash the eggs with a fork. Add salt and pepper to taste and serve with the hot toast.

Ham And Eggs

Ingredients:

- 1 tbsp. butter (or a non-dairy version)

- Ketchup (13g is a low FODMAP portion) – optional

- 1 egg

- 50g smoked cooked ham

- 1 gluten-free crumpet or muffin

Directions:

1. Put your crumpet or muffin in the toaster and while it's toasting fry your egg.
2. When your egg is almost done put the ham in the frying pan to heat through.

3. Once your crumpet/muffin is toasted put it on
    a plate and butter it.
4. Place the ham on top followed by the fried
    egg and season to taste before serving.

Low Fodmap Salad

Ingredients:

- 1 small carrot ribboned with a potato pealer

- 3 radishes thinly sliced

- 1 handful of olives

- oz | 65g common tomato or strawberries

- 1.7 oz | 50g pickled beetroot

- oz | 100g butter, iceberg or red coral lettuce OR a mix of the 3

- 1.7 oz | 50g arugula/rocket lettuce

- 1/3 cucumber

- oz | 100g grilled chicken breast OR leftover chicken OR a boiled egg OR a can of tuna

- 3 tbsp chives cut with scissors

For the salad dressing

- 3 tbsp olive oil extra virgin

- 1 tbsp red wine vinegar OR apple cider vinegar

- Salt and black pepper to taste

Directions:

Make the salad dressing

1. Place all ingredients in a mason jar, put the lid on and shake well until completely mixed.
2. Store the sauce in the jar in the refrigerator and use it only when eating the salad.

Make the salad

1. Place all the ingredients in a large bowl or in a lunch box with a lid.
2. Store in the refrigerator covered until you eat.

3. Before serving, pour the dressing over the
    salad and mix well. Eat immediately.

Low Fodmap Tuna Salad

Ingredients:

Tahini dressing

- 1 tbsp water

- 1/4 tsp salt

- 1/2 tsp dried dill

- 1 tbsp tahini

- 1.5 tbsp red wine vinegar

- 0.5 tbsp dijon mustard

Tuna salad

- 1 can tuna, drained

- 1/4 cup cucumber, chopped

- 2-3 tbsp green onion (green part only)

Directions:

1. Start by mixting together all the dressing ingredients in the bottom of the bowl you plan on making the tuna salad in. Stir well until fully combined.
2. Next drain the tuna and add it to the bowl with the dressing.
3. Chop the cucumber and slice the green onion. Add the veggies to the tuna in the bowl.
4. Stir well, breaking up the tuna as needed. Taste for salt and serve your favorite way!

Caramelized Pork Tacos With Pineapple Salsa

Ingredients:

For the pork:

- 1 tablespoon oil

- 1 shallot, minced

- 1 clove garlic, minced

- 1 jalapeño, diced with ribs and seeds removed

- 2 teaspoons fish sauce

- 18 ounces boneless pork loin, sliced into thin strips

- 2 tablespoons sugar

- 2 tablespoons water

For the pineapple salsa

- 1 cup chopped pineapple

- 1 cup chopped cucumber

- 1/2 cup chopped cilantro

- 1/2 cup chopped red onion or shallot

- A squeeze of lime juice

- A pinch of salt

- Tortillas for serving

- Cilantro and lime for serving

- Chili sauce for topping – see notes

Directions:

1. **For The Pork**: Heat the oil in a heavy pan over medium heat. Add the shallot, garlic, and

jalapeño – saute until fragrant, about 2
minutes. Turn the heat to high and add the
pork and the fish sauce – stir fry for a few
minutes until the pork is no longer pink. With
the heat very high, add the sugar and water
and stir once – then let the pork caramelize by
not stirring it for about 1 minute. Repeat this
process until the pork is nice and golden
brown.

2. **For The Salsa:** Toss everything together in a
medium bowl.

3. **For The Tacos**: Warm the tortillas quickly in a
skillet with a little bit of oil. Arrange the pork
between 6 tortillas and top with the salsa and
the chili sauce.

Vietnamese Rice Noodle Bowl

Ingredients:

- 1 head of green leaf lettuce, washed, dried, and torn into large pieces

- 1 cup of cilantro

- 1 cup of mint

- 1/4 cup tamari almonds, roughly chopped

- 1 package, 8.8 ounce of brown rice vermicelli noodles, cooked according to package

- 2 persian cucumbers, thinly sliced

- 4 radishes, thinly sliced

Quick pickled veggies

- 1 daikon radish, julienned

- Rice wine vinegar, unsweetened

- Dash of honey

- 2 carrots, julienned

- Pinch of salt

Dressing

- 1/4 cup lime juice

- 2 tablespoon fresh orange juice

- 2 tablespoons rice wine vinegar

- 2 tablespoon low-sodium gluten free tamari

- 1 tablespoon raw honey

- 2 tablespoons sesame oil

- 1 serrano chili, thinly sliced

Directions:

1. Combine carrots and daikon in a small bowl and toss with rice wine vinegar, a dash of honey and salt. Set aside while you prep your other vegetables.

2. Whisk all ingredients together for dressing and set aside.

3. Assemble bowls by places a few pieces of lettuce at the bottom on the bowls and topping with the noodles, cucumbers, radish, cilantro, mint, almonds and pickled vegetables.

4. Top each bowl with a few tablespoons of dressing, mix well and enjoy!

5. Feel free to add steamed edamame, pan fried tofu or grilled shrimp for an extra punch of protein.

Spicy Potato Pie - Low Fodmap And Gluten-Free

Ingredients:

- 1 tbsp cooking oil

- 1 red pepper, chopped finely

- 6 rashers of bacon

- 1 bag of baby spinach leaves, chopped into fine strips

- 4 eggs

- ⅓ cup rice flour and tapioca flour mixed

- 4 large potatoes

- 3 spring onions (green part only), sliced up

- 1 red chilli, finely chopped

- 2 tsp garlic-infused oil

- Salt and pepper

Directions:

1. Heat oven to 180°C/350°F.
2. Heat the two oils and cook the chilli and spring onions until soft.
3. Add the bacon and cook, then chop into hunks.
4. Peel and grate the potatoes. Squeeze out all excess liquid.
5. Mix all ingredients together.
6. Oil a tart pan and tip the mixture in and flatten the top.
7. Bake in the oven for about 30 minutes.

Kale And Olive Pasta

Ingredients:

- 1 sundried tomato

- 2 tbsp of pumpkin seeds

- Salt and pepper

- 1 tbsp of pitted black olives

- 1 tbsp of uncooked tomato puree

- 1 tsp of garlic-infused oil

- 1 tsp of balsamic vinegar

- 1 large saucepan

- 1 large frying pan

- 70 g of gluten-free pasta uncooked

- 46 g of canned green lentils

- 2 full handfuls of kale (you can use more or less depending on your tastes)

- 2-3 common tomatoes

Directions:

1. Begin by heating water in your large saucepan. Once it comes to a boil, add in a little salt for flavor, and then place your gluten-free pasta.
2. Let the pasta cook according to the package directions.
3. Place your large frying pan over a medium flame and pour in your sunflower seeds so that they begin to toast.
4. This should be done while the seeds and your pan are dry.

5. Once the seeds begin to give off a nutty aroma and start popping in the pan, add your drained and rinsed lentils.

6. Stir the seeds and lentils together for a minute or two and then add chopped kale and sliced tomatoes to the pan.

7. You might need to add some water to the pan so that the kale reduces as it cooks and doesn't burn.

8. Once the kale has begun to cook down, stir in your finely chopped sundried tomato, black olives, balsamic vinegar, garlic-infused oil, and tomato puree and let everything cook together. As you stir the sauce, add in little bits of water if you need to thin down the sauce or help it cooks.

9. Heat and stir the sauce until it begins to smush together.

10. Your sauce should be done by the time your pasta is done cooking in the pot. At this point,

add the cooked pasta into the large frying pan with the sauce and stir everything together to combine it evenly.

11. To finish, serve your pasta dish in a large bowl with a sprinkle of pepper or salt to your liking. Enjoy!

Chinese Noodle Soup

Ingredients:

- 2 cups of a low-FODMAP vegetable stock

- 1 full nest of rice noodles

- ¼ tsp of turmeric

- 2 tbsp of green onions/scallions (only use green part)

- 2 tsp of ginger root

- 1 tbsp soy sauce

- 1 tsp corn starch or cornflour

- 1 tsp miso paste

- 1 large saucepan

- 100 g of firm tofu

- 1 large tomato

- 1 sheet of Nori (seaweed sheet)

- 1 tbsp sesame oil

Directions:

1. Chop your tofu into small, bite-sized chunks, and chop the Nori sheet into small flakes. Peel the ginger root and then make sure to dice both the tomato and the ginger root finely.

2. Set your saucepan over medium heat, heat half the sesame oil in the pot, and then add in your tofu chunks. Place your turmeric powder, finely chopped ginger, and half of your soy sauce over the tofu. Once it has begun to warm up, stir in your miso paste and finely diced tomatoes. Add salt and pepper to taste.

3. As this tofu mixture continues to heat up, pour in the vegetable stock and break the rice noodles into it. Let the noodles soften in the vegetable stock for about 2–3 minutes and then sprinkle in the Nori flakes.

4. In a separate small bowl, mix your corn starch or cornflour with about 2 tbsp of water. Pour this mixture into the noodle soup that you are cooking in your pot, and begin to stir the soup very fast. Continue to stir as the soup begins to thicken.

5. Serve in a bowl. Pour the rest of the sesame oil and soy sauce over the soup. Finally, season the soup with your green onions and black pepper and enjoy!

Spinach And Tofu Plate Of Mixed Greens

Ingredients:

- ½ cup ground carrot

- 2 teaspoons sesame seeds

- 2 teaspoons lemon squeeze (or dressing of decision)

- 2 cups child spinach

- ½ cup firm cooked tofu

Directions:

1. Spot child spinach in a bowl.
2. Include sesame seeds and blend well to guarantee seeds have spread equitably among the child spinach leaves.

3. Include ground carrot, tofu and lemon juice (or other dressing) and blend once more.
4. Refrigerate (spinach plate of mixed greens ought to be served cold).

Vanilla Chia Pudding

Ingredients:

- 2 tablespoon maple syrup or agave 1 teaspoon vanilla concentrate

- 1/2 teaspoon cinnamon

- 6 tablespoons chia seeds 2 cups almond milk

Directions:

1. Blend up the almond milk, vanilla, maple syrup, and cinnamon.
2. Pour fluid blend over the chia seeds and mix till seeds are equally blended in.
3. Mix again five minutes after the fact, and five minutes after that.
4. Let sit for an hour at any rate, or essentially let it sit in the cooler medium-term.
5. Serve; beat with crisp product of decision.

6. Pudding will keep in the refrigerator for as

    long as four days.

Tasty Egg Wraps

Ingredients:

- 41 grams eggplant, sliced

- 1/8 teaspoon paprika

- ½ red bell pepper, deseeded and sliced

- 66 grams zucchini, grated

- 70 grams carrot, grated

- 1 ½ tablespoon mayonnaise

- ½ teaspoon lemon juice

- 2 large eggs

- ½ tablespoon plain flour, gluten-free

- 1 ½ tablespoon almond milk

- ½ teaspoon garlic-infused oil

- Salt and pepper

- Canola oil

Directions:

1. Place almond milk and flour in a bowl. Mix well.
2. Whisk in eggs and season to taste.
3. Pour a serving of the mixture into a pan and cook in canola oil for a minute. Flip the egg wrap and cook for another 30 seconds. Do the same step for the remaining mixture.
4. Fry eggplant and bell pepper over medium-high flame for 4 minutes. Add zucchini and carrots and cook for another 3 minutes. Sprinkle paprika, salt and pepper.
5. Place mayonnaise, lemon juice and garlic-infused oil in a bowl and mix well. Sprinkle black pepper over the mixture.

6. Arrange an egg wrap in a plate. Place the cooked vegetables in the middle and drizzle with mayonnaise mixture. Roll the egg wrap around the filling.

Purple Breakfast Smoothie

Ingredients:

- 1 tablespoon peanut butter

- ¾ cup almond milk

- 4 ice cubes

- ½ banana, sliced

- ½ cup blueberries

Directions:

1. Place all of the ingredients in a blender.
2. Process until smooth.

Chinese Eggplant

Ingredients:

- 1 ½ tablespoons gluten-free soy sauce (tamari)

- 1 tablespoon gluten-free fish sauce

- 1/16 teaspoon wheat-free asafetida powder

- 2 teaspoons turbinado sugar

- 1 1/2 tablespoons sesame oil

- 1 teaspoon minced (fresh or dry) ginger

- 1 pound (or 2) Chinese (long) eggplant, sliced into quarters

- 1/4 teaspoon salt

- 1 teaspoon cornstarch, plus ¼ cup more to coat eggplant

- 1 tablespoon safflower oil

- 3 scallions, chopped, green tips only

Directions:

1. Spread sliced eggplant on a paper towel and sprinkle salt on both sides of eggplant slices. Allow to rest for 1 hour to draw the water out of the eggplant. Pat eggplant dry but do not rinse.

2. Combine soy sauce, fish sauce, asafetida powder, sugar and 1 teaspoon cornstarch in a bowl and mix well.

3. Sprinkle ¼ cup cornstarch over the eggplant until the eggplant is evenly coated. Add more cornstarch if needed to coat both sides evenly, making sure each piece of the eggplant is coated.

4. Heat the oil in a non-stick skillet. Add in ginger and 2 chopped scallions and the sauce. Place eggplant across the surface of the skillet and do not overlap pieces. Grill eggplant pieces until charred and soft, about 8 -10 minutes per side. Transfer to a plate.

Classic Roast Beef Withvegetables

Ingredients:

- 1.5kg (about 10) white potatoes, peeled, halved lengthways, patted dry with paper towel

- 2 bunches baby carrots, trimmed to 1cm, washed, scrubbed, patted dry with paper towel

- 1 tablespoon gluten-free flour

- 375ml (1 1/2 cups) Campbell's

- 2 tablespoons butter, at room temperature

- 6 teaspoons olive oil

- 1 2kg rib eye roast

- Salt & freshly ground black pepper

- Beef Real Stock

- Steamed spinach or green beans, to serve

Directions:

1. Preheat oven to 425F. Heat 2 teaspoons of the butter and 2 teaspoons oil in a large shallow skillet over high heat. Cook the roast, turning occasionally, for 5 minutes or until well browned.

2. Remove skillet from heat and season beef all over with salt and pepper.

3. Place the potatoes, 3 teaspoons of the remaining butter and 1 teaspoon of the remaining oil in a bowl. Put disposable gloves on your hands (you will thank me later!) and use your hands to rub the butter and oil evenly over the potatoes. Season the

potatoes with salt and pepper. Arrange the potatoes in a single layer around the beef.

4. Cook beef and potatoes in the preheated oven for 30 minutes, basting beef with the pan juices once during cooking to keep the beef moist.

5. Place remaining oil and butter in another roasting pan or roasting skillet. Place this pan in the oven for 5 minutes or until butter melts. Add carrots and toss the carrots in the butter to coat well. Turn the potatoes and baste the beef in their roaster. Now add the carrots to the oven and cook, shaking the carrot pan occasionally, for 25 minutes or until the beef is medium or cooked to your liking.

6. Transfer beef to a large plate and cover loosely with foil. Set aside for 15 minutes to rest. While beef is resting, transfer the potatoes to a tray lined with aluminum foil.

Increase oven temperature to 475F. Return potatoes to oven and continue to cook while beef is resting. To make gravy, strain pan juices from the roasting pan into a heatproof container. Return 2 tablespoons of pan juices to a saucepan and heat over high heat. Mix the flour with hot water until it makes a smooth paste. Add this paste to the broth/juices and stir. Cook until thickens, constantly stirring.

7. Gradually add the stock and cook, scraping the pan with a wooden spoon to dislodge any bits cooked onto the base of the pan.

8. Slice the beef across the grain and serve with the gravy, roast potatoes, roast carrots and steamed spinach or beans.

9. Add crusty rolls and a tasty dessert for a special family meal.